QUICK EASY yoga

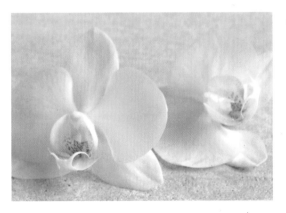

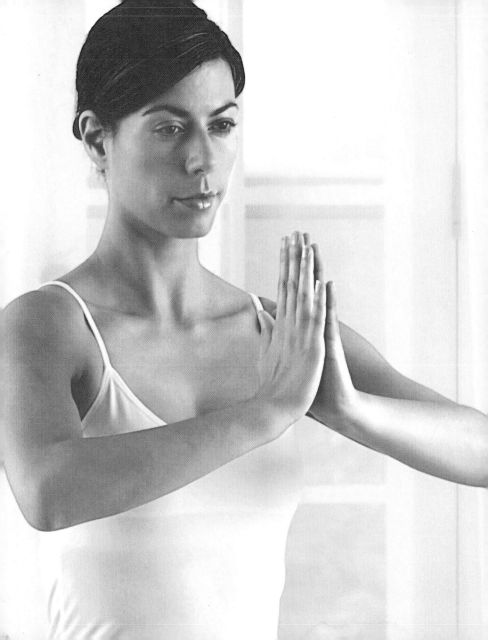

DUNCAN BAIRD PUBLISHERS

LONDON

QUICK & EASY yoga

Christina Brown

5-minute routines for

anyone

anytime

anywhere

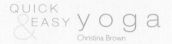

QUICK
& EASY yoga
Christina Brown

Distributed in the USA and Canada by
Sterling Publishing Co., Inc.
387 Park Avenue South, New York, NY 10016-8810

This edition first published in the UK in 2008 and in the USA in 2009 by
Duncan Baird Publishers Ltd
Sixth Floor, Castle House, 75–76 Wells Street, London W1T 3QH

Managing Editor: Grace Cheetham
Editor: Zoë Fargher
Managing Designer: Manisha Patel
Designer: Jantje Doughty
Commissioned photography: Jules Selmes

Library of Congress Cataloging-in-Publication Data

Brown, Christina.
   Quick & easy yoga : 5 minute routines for anyone, anytime, anywhere / Christina
Brown.
     p. cm.
   Includes index.
   ISBN 978-1-84483-838-7
   1. Hatha yoga. I. Title. II. Title: Quick and easy yoga.
   RA781.7.B758 2009
   613.7046--dc22

                                        2009000861

ISBN: 978-1-84483-838-7
10 9 8 7 6 5 4 3 2 1

Typeset in Gill Sans, Nofret and Helvetica Neue
Color reproduction by Scanhouse, Malaysia
Printed in China by Imago

For information about custom editions, special sales, premium and corporate
purchases, please contact Sterling Special Sales Department at 800-805-5489
or specialsales@sterlingpub.com.

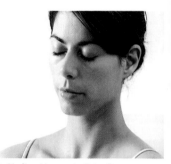

To Nadine Uremovic, Peter Ross,
and Kristy Lee McMullen for
supporting the writing process,
and to all my teachers.

contents

introduction

According to the Oxford English Dictionary committee, the most commonly used noun in the English language is "time". We spend time, watch time, manage time, keep time and lose time, but most of all, it seems, we're trying to save time. We feel that we haven't enough of it. With all this emphasis on efficiency in our modern world, it makes sense to find quick and effective ways to relax, too. Although a yoga practice can last hours, it is possible to feel the benefits in minutes. This book is intended to eliminate the oft-heard excuse, "I don't have time for yoga", and offer simple, speedy exercises that will revive, rejuvenate and restore you in as little as five minutes.

My students often enter class hurried and harried or else lethargic and low in energy. But within the first five minutes of class, I can see them shift into bliss mode. The truth is, you don't need to hide away in a cave in the Himalayas or dedicate years of your life solely to yoga to enjoy its benefits. You can begin to welcome the joys of yoga into your life by simply dipping into this book for five, ten or 20 minutes, and practising one or more exercises.

why is yoga so good for us?

Yoga postures strengthen, lengthen, limber and loosen our bodies, energize, calm, focus and purify our minds, and build stamina and suppleness in our muscles, tendons and ligaments. Hatha Yoga (postures combined with breathing and meditation, as featured in this book) is an ideal form of exercise if you lead a sedentary lifestyle. Many of us leave work only to commute home, eat dinner and watch television, all in the same seated position we've been in all day, with our shoulders hunched and our backs rolled forward. Even household duties such as washing dishes, vacuuming, ironing, cooking and cleaning make us slump. Yoga postures are incredibly helpful for people who sit at a desk in front of a computer for most of their day, or whose other daily tasks negatively affect their posture. When each day risks looking like a series of slouchy forward bends, our bodies yearn for side stretches, twists and backbends, and they rejoice when we practise them.

Yoga practice also rounds us out. Modern life places huge importance on the intellect, and yoga brings a fresh awareness if we've lost touch with our physical selves. I have watched students who were stiff and stressed at the start of a class float off lithely down the street afterward, and after a single class, people tell me that they stand taller and sleep better. The wholesome discipline of yoga just makes life feel better and easier. Yoga practice is a doubly rewarding – it may be part of your inner journey toward harmony, but the practice feels so good physically, it is also a reward in itself.

mind, body and soul

Most people know that yoga practice counteracts the asymmetry and bad postural habits of our physical bodies. But Hatha Yoga is unique compared to other forms of exercise, because it reaches out to all aspects of our being. Yoga touches our minds, our hearts and our souls, reuniting body, breath, mind, emotions and spirit. You'll know this if you've ever relaxed deeply at the end of a yoga class, or let yourself release into a soft, nurturing yoga pose, or flooded your body with consciousness in an energetic, enlivening stretch. Inner peace comes as you relax back into a sense of wholeness. It's like a long sigh out as you sink back in a warm bath at the end of a long day. It's when you remember who you really are when, caught up in the whirlwind of life, you had forgotten. As so many people have discovered, the practice of a single, simple posture can set your mind at ease and make your heart sing. For this reason, people all over the world have fallen in love with yoga and reaped its rewards.

Yoga is also a state of mind. The word yoga can be translated as the cessation of the fluctuations in the mind – we are in the state of yoga when our mind is still. The physical practices of yoga were developed to keep our bodies healthy, while the breathing and meditative practices were honed to guide our minds into the experience of this state of

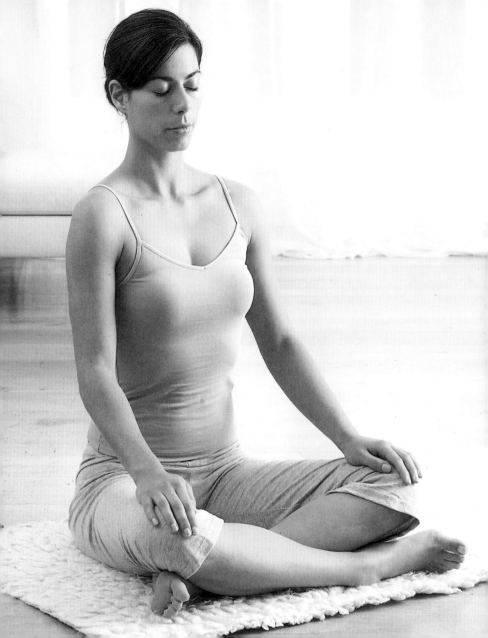

yoga. You may simply choose to enjoy the physical benefits of your posture practice – that's fine. But, should you choose to go further, the rich yogic philosophy originating from India dates back 2,000 years, and contains the answers to key questions that have been pondered throughout human history: who am I? Why am I here? Ultimately, you can achieve self-realization with the help of yoga.

Many of us seek these answers outside of ourselves, forgetting that we hold them within. The sequences in this book are designed to strengthen, ease and release the body and to start you off on your journey of self-discovery. We often think that to improve we need to go deeper, longer, stronger or harder, and we expend a lot of effort in the struggle to get to an imagined space, where all our troubles magically fall away. But sometimes getting "better" is actually about just "being". Consider that you don't have to "go" anywhere to come home to yourself. Eventually you'll come to know that you've already arrived. Try being content right now, right where you are, and see if you can adopt this way of thinking during your yoga practice.

In the first two chapters of this book are five-minute exercises you can practise anytime and anywhere you can find a moment and a little space. Of course, you don't have to practise the exercise entitled "at work" there and then – you could try it in the bus queue, or while you're waiting at a supermarket checkout. Be creative, and it'll be even easier to enjoy your yoga practice and adapt it to your life.

I've also tailored specific exercises to be Stress Busters, Mood Enhancers or Energy Boosters, and these make up the next three chapters. The final chapter contains exercises to practise with a partner: this can be a great way to bond with a loved one, and may make it easier to absorb yoga into your daily routine. Finally, if you have a little longer to practise, at the back of this book I've included a selection of everyday sequences. These will take between 30 minutes and an hour each to complete, and are the ideal way to start a home practice.

as you practise

The key to the effectiveness of yoga is where you place your focus during your practice. If you observe your thoughts for just a few minutes, you will notice that they rarely stay in the present moment, or on a single object. They tend to move to either the past or the future, and there to spin in endless circles.

During your yoga practice, try to bring your attention to your breath and your body. Both of these can exist only in the present moment – it is impossible for them to exist yesterday or tomorrow, in the past or in the future. Focusing on either your breath or body will bring your mind back to right here, right now. It elevates your mind away from its usual preoccupations, and allows a shift in consciousness to occur. In this mode of being, we can enter a state of easy flow, where our daily stresses drop away and we are lifted up and out of our usual limiting thought patterns.

If you are completely new to yoga, you may require a little time to enter this "flow" state. You may find it easier in a calm environment or when your mind is already fairly quiet. However, with practice, a single yoga posture from this book can take you there, and eventually you'll find that you can reach this special state of being quite quickly, in less than ideal circumstances or even when your mind is agitated. You don't need to experience this flow state for long periods of time to increase your general contentment levels. Dipping into it even briefly can radically improve the quality of your day.

Sometimes you'll find you'll begin your practice feeling restless, tight, anxious and finding it hard to focus. Or sometimes you may start on the other extreme, feeling heavy, sleepy, lazy and lethargic. The important thing is to begin, and trust that your yoga practice will ease you back into balance. After absorbing yourself in your practice, you may well finish feeling warmer, looser, calmer, more relaxed, and perhaps more connected to a helpful force greater than you.

breathing

There is an intrinsic link between our breath and our minds – a change in one will inevitably affect the other. When you feel restless and unsettled, focusing on the breath is reassuring, soothing and healing. When you feel sleepy and dull, breathing consciously can be cleansing and clarifying and bring freshness your day.

Always breathe in and out through your nose so that your breath is filtered and warmed (mouth breathing is used only very occasionally in yoga). In general, inhale when you are opening or unfolding your body, when you are rising up or lengthening, when twisting your upper back and when bending backward. Exhale when releasing, closing your body, moving downward, twisting your lower back, lowering your arms or legs, and when bending forward or sideways. Stay in tune with what feels right for you as you move, and bear in mind that even in postures where your body looks still, your breath is always moving.

find your edge

Your yoga practice should always bring you joy and enhance your life. If your practice is too intense or painful, your body and mind will clench up and pull away from it. Conversely, if you are underworking, your body and mind will both get bored. Work on finding that optimum

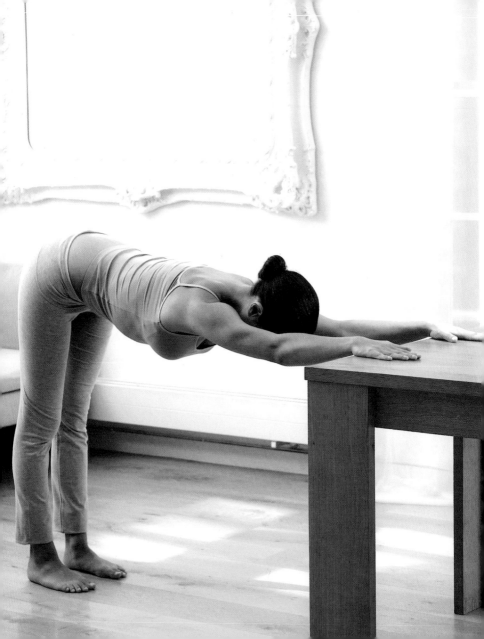

point – your edge. Finding your edge means that you will be working with a healthy amount of tension, yet you will still be able to experience quietness and relaxation in the exercise.

Keep in mind that the intensity you may feel in a strong stretch is not necessarily bad. Pain is more acute than discomfort, and there will be nothing pleasant about it. If you do feel pain in a pose, it means that you are improperly aligned or that you are pushing yourself too far. Ignoring pain could lead to injury, so come out of that exercise and check with an experienced yoga teacher.

To work more gently, ensure that you rest well between exercises. Practise poses such as those on page 56 or 64 whenever you feel the need. Check often that you are breathing calmly. Move slowly from pose to pose and relax your muscles in each posture. Keep your face and eyes relaxed. Pay attention to basic instructions on alignment, such as where your knees and toes should point. Try not to hunch your shoulders, particularly when raising your arms. Bend your knees when leaning forward, or when coming up from a forward bend to standing.

building up sequences

As many exercises in this book are creative combinations of yoga postures, they work as stand-alone practices. However, if you would like to try to build up your own sequences, aim to include all of the following: a twisting movement, a side stretch, a forward bend, a backbend, a balance, an abdominal strengthener, an inversion, and a soft, centering pose. The six sequences at the back of this book will help to get you started on a home yoga practice.

on meditation

Generally, people associate yoga with the practice of postures (*asana*). These postures naturally concentrate the mind, bringing it into a more meditative space. While your motivation to begin regular *asana* practice may have been to tone your muscles or cure a bad back, you may be pleasantly surprised by the positive mental effects regular yoga offers.

Classically the aim of a yoga practice (and, as I've said, the definition of the word yoga) is to quiet the movements of the mind, and you may find you touch this quietening while practising the exercises in this book. People often imagine meditation to be about achieving one specific state of mind. But meditation is a journey, not an endpoint. The best thing you can do is observe and try to enjoy the process. Learn to smile tenderly at yourself if you find yourself getting frustrated or uptight. Let go of having to attain anything. When you do, you will find that you're happier with your practice and happier with yourself in

16

general. Plus, you'll notice a funny thing: you'll find that regardless of your opinion of the quality of your performance of the poses, your day will feel sunnier when you've practised yoga.

practice tips

Finally, here are a few practical suggestions to help you find more enjoyment in your particular experience of yoga:

Don't worry about your flexibility. If you can breathe, you can practise yoga. People often say to me that they are not flexible enough for yoga. The thing is, you don't need to start off flexible to become flexible! The poses in this book are suitable for even the stiffest of people. It's often the stiffer-bodied among us who notice results first – I have seen remarkable improvements in students in just four sessions.

Do fit your practices in where you can. I delayed sitting down to meditate for years because I believed my house had to be perfectly clean before I could relax into my practice – and I mean the whole house! Neither housework nor many other tasks in our daily lives are ever really finished, and there will always something more you can use as an excuse to put off your dedication to your health and happiness. So, whatever sticking point you have, drop it now, and commit afresh to your health and well-being.

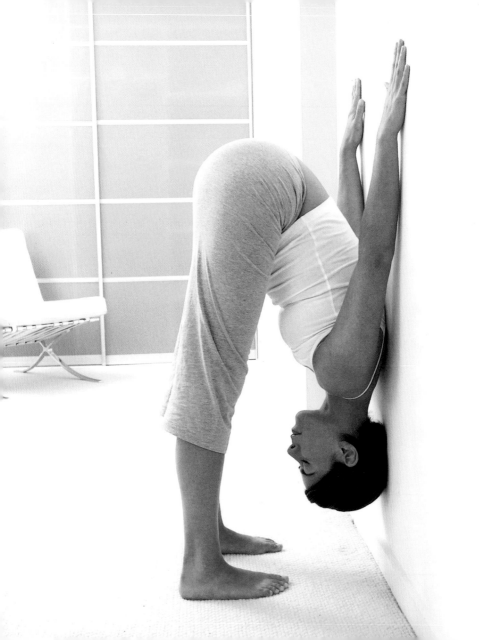

Do wear comfortable, stretchy clothes that you feel good in, and remove shoes and socks. If you don't have a fabric yoga belt like those used in classes, use a strip of material such as a bathrobe tie.

Do try to practise on an empty stomach. If you can, leave three hours after a big meal, and an hour after a light meal. If you are planning a longer practice, drink plenty of water 30 minutes before you begin, so you won't need to rehydrate as you practise.

Most importantly, if you have an injury or illness, or if you are pregnant, get clearance from your health professional before practising any of these exercises and seek advice from an experienced teacher.

Yoga has given me so much pleasure over the years and I hope it brings you joy too. Many people never get around to starting yoga because they feel they are too busy; this book is intended to encourage you to bring yoga into your life in as many small ways as possible. Creating little pockets of time for yourself will lift your general level of contentment beyond what you may expect. Enjoy these spaces, come back to your centre and open into a dialogue with yourself. Be aware that yoga isn't about self-improvement at the cost of self-acceptance. Rather than just seeking to touch your toes, remind yourself that practising yoga is also about touching your own heart.

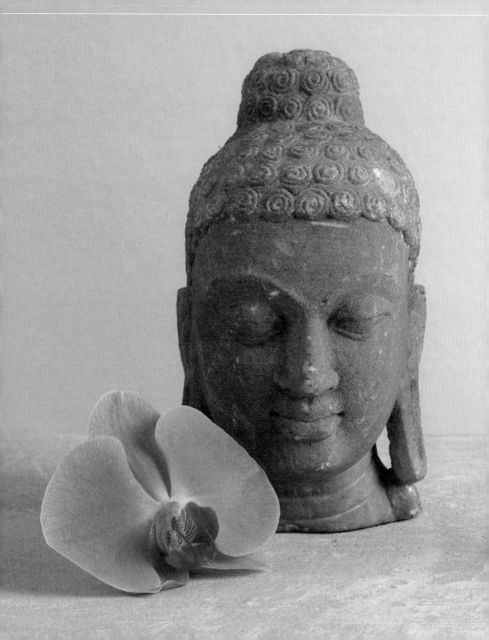

anytime

Greet the morning with an invigorating yoga sequence or enhance

your well-being during the day with a mini lunchtime practice. Yoga

techniques work anytime, whether you need to refresh and refocus

before a long meeting, or soothe yourself to get ready for sleep.

1

Kneel with your knees together. Fold at your hips, and reach your arms forward, hands shoulder-width apart. Spread your palms broadly, and send the muscle activation through your arm muscles to press your buttocks toward your heels. This position is your start and end point.

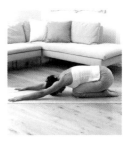

2

As you inhale, lift your shoulders to exactly above your wrists. Position your hips so that your neck and spine form a straight line between your knees and your shoulders. Ensure your inner elbow creases face forward, and point your toes straight up to the sky.

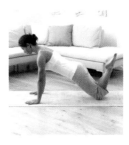

3

(*right*) On your next exhalation, bend your elbows to hover your chest above the floor. Pull your elbows back so that they graze your side-ribs, rather than bending out to the sides. Draw your navel to your spine to activate your abdominal muscles so there is no sagging in your back.

4

On your next inhalation, press back up to place your shoulders above your wrists. To prevent your back sagging, engage your abdominal muscles. Finally, as you exhale, return to your start position. Guided by your breath, complete four more cycles of this four-step sequence.

morning activator
invigorating

let your breath guide you through flowing movements

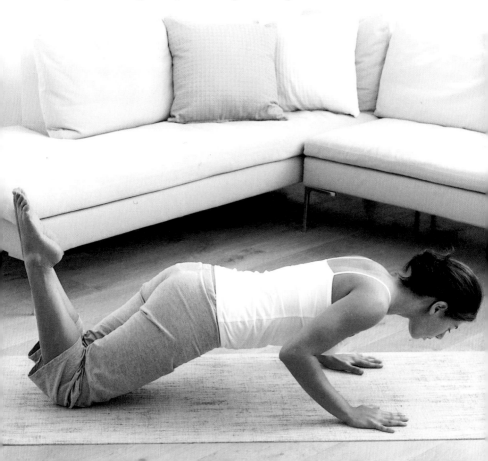

1 Sit on the floor and bend your right knee back so that your right foot nestles in toward your right buttock. Take the sole of your left foot to rest under your right inner thigh. Interlace your fingers and take them behind your head. Keep both buttocks anchored to the floor.

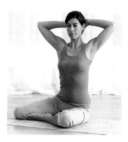

2 (*right*) Inhale and spread your inner elbows wide as your chest expands. Then exhale and, keeping your elbows broad, twist to your left. Allow your right hipbone to travel with you into this twist so it moves forward and up. Let your abdomen squeeze inward and swivel to the left, too.

3 Inhale and return to your starting position. Feel both your buttocks pressing evenly into the floor. Take your time; don't rush your inhalation, and be aware of how the centre of your chest lifts as you breathe in. Enjoy this energizing part of your breath.

4 On your next exhalation, drop your right elbow toward your right foot. Actively extend your left elbow upward while lifting and spreading your left side-ribs. Inhale to return to centre, and repeat the twist and sideways stretch five times, inhaling to twist, and exhaling to stretch. Then swap your leg positions to practise on the other side.

get up and go
energizing

awaken your core
to enliven your day

mid-morning wake-up
uplifting

recharge with this energetic sequence

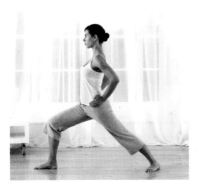 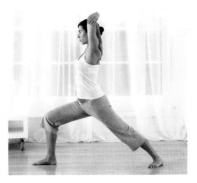

1 Stand with your feet about 1.5m (5ft) apart and your hands on your hips. Point your right toes straight forward and the toes of your left foot out at a 45-degree angle. Move your left hip forward so your hips are square to the front. Bend your front leg so your knee joint sits just above your ankle.

2 Reach up with your left arm. Rotating your shoulder internally, swivel your arm so your thumb points behind you. Bend your elbow and drop your hand behind your head, reaching as far down your back as possible. Cup your left elbow in your right hand to increase the stretch.

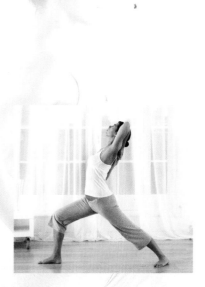

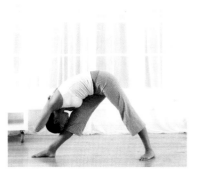

3 Stay here or, for a deeper shoulder stretch, take your right arm behind your back and nudge your hand up to grasp your left fingers (or hold a belt between your hands). Gaze up and use the pressure of your hands snuggling into your spine to bring you into a gentle backbend.

4 Exhale as you straighten your front knee and fold at your hips into a deep forward bend. Then inhale, bend your knee and come back to your backbend. Move between these two positions; upward on each inhalation and forward on each exhalation. After ten breaths, practise on the other side.

27

1 Stand with your feet hip-width apart. Take your arms overhead, palms facing each other. Slide your shoulder blades down your back so your neck feels long and free. Press your feet firmly into the floor and slide your knees forward so that you are in a gentle squat. Arch your spine.

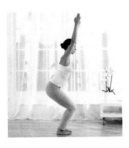

2 After six breaths, bring your palms together at your chest. Push your palms together strongly and feel your chest muscles engage. Check that your knees are in line with your middle toes, which point straight forward. Maintain the activation in your back muscles.

3 (*right*) Now squat deeper as you twist and take your left elbow to rest against your right outer knee. Open your elbows a little more so that your wrists are close to your chest. See if you can realign your knees so they are level. Turn your head to look up for eight breaths.

4 Return to your symmetrical starting position. Again take your arms overhead, palms facing each other, and imagine your arms are an extension of your spine, allowing it to elongate. Hold for five breaths to re-centre. Then twist to the other side. Rotate your trunk to the left and bring your right elbow to the left outer knee as you look up past the left shoulder. Release back to centre after eight breaths..

lunchtime lift
balancing

clear your mind with
a re-centering twist

afternoon stabilizer releasing

ease out the tensions of a long day

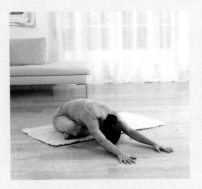

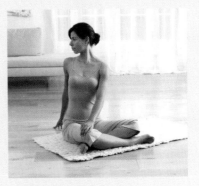

1 Sit in a cross-legged position, breathe in and reach both arms up. As you exhale, reach out through the front of your torso to bring both hands to the floor in front of you. Inhale and exhale six times to gradually slide your chest forward. Then release your neck and stay here for ten breaths.

2 Inhale to come up. Bring your left hand to your right knee, and your right fingertips to the floor behind you. Find a spot that gives you the best traction for a strong twist, and twist to the right. Inhale and grow taller. As you exhale, narrow your waist and intensify the twist. Stay here for five breaths.

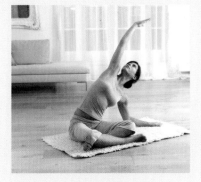 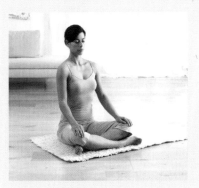

3 Return to centre. Slide your left hand along the floor, in line with your hip. Extend your right arm up and over to the left, palm facing down, into a long, enjoyable side stretch. Reach actively to develop a strong, smooth line. Stay here for five breaths. Change the way your legs are crossed, and repeat the whole sequence on the other side.

4 Now place your hands on your knees, float your spine tall, and feel buoyant in your chest. With your eyes closed, stay in this position, observing your breathing for ten slow breaths. Stay connected to that peaceful space within, as you slowly open your eyes to greet the world outside.

evening
de-stress
restoring

feel the full weight of gravity
to help you relax deeply

1

Lie on your back with your knees bent in. Hold your knees and slowly circle them clockwise five times, giving your lower back a soothing massage. Change direction to circle the knees anti-clockwise. Then, hug your knees tighter into your chest and slowly rock from side to side to release tension in your whole back.

2

Drape your right arm around both shins and take your left arm out to the side, hand level with your shoulders. Squeeze both knees in, then bring them over to the right, so they are snuggled in as close to your armpit as possible. Release your left shoulder toward the floor, and extend your right arm out to the side.

3

(*left*) Completely relax both legs to the floor. Make sure your ankles and feet feel floppy. Allow your shoulder blades to broaden across your back. Turn your head to the left. There is no more work to do in this pose. Just relax, breathe evenly, feel your face soften and let your skin feel smooth as butter. Enjoy.

4

After two minutes, lift your legs to return to the centre. Lie flat and notice how your lower back feels. Observe how the left side of your lower back feels flatter, longer, looser and happier! Even yourself up with a leisurely twist to the left side, then finish with five more knee circles, clockwise and anti-clockwise.

33

1   Fold up a blanket and place it on the seat of a chair. Sit on the floor with your legs straight out, between the legs of the chair, which should be about 60cm (2ft) in front of you. Bend your right knee outward, to bring the sole of your right foot to rest against your left inner thigh.

2   Inhale, raise your arms and as you exhale, fold forward to drape your arms over the seat of the chair. Allow your forehead to rest on the blanket at the front edge of the chair. You may need to fold the blanket again so that your forehead can reach its resting spot comfortably.

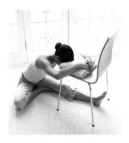

3   (*right*) If you are very flexible, place a folded blanket on your straight leg and bend forward to rest your forehead on it. Whether you choose this or the previous version, stay here for two minutes, breathing deeply. As you surrender into the posture, you can slide the chair or blankets away from you to increase the stretch. Repeat on the other side.

4   For an enjoyable variation, take your legs into a wide V-shape. Place the chair in the middle and fold toward it. Drape your arms loosely over the seat of the chair and support your forehead on the blanket. Close your eyes and rest here for two minutes or more. As your body releases, nudge the chair forward to increase the stretch.

bedtime wind-down
nurturing
turn your back on the outer world and relax your inner world

close the day
soothing

soften shoulder tension
and lay your worries down

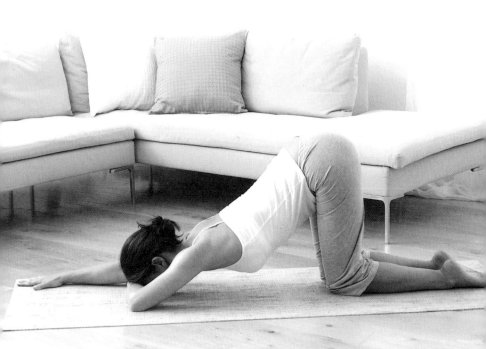

1 From an all-fours position, bring both forearms to the floor. Reach your right palm forward along the floor as far as you can. Slide your left palm under your right elbow. Check that your hips are directly above your knee joints, to ensure you fully appreciate the deep lengthening this posture offers.

2 Keeping your right elbow off the floor, energetically reach forward with your right palm and lower your forehead to your left forearm. Check again that your hips are over your knees, and walk your knees backward to correct this if necessary.

3 Play around with the position of your left forearm so that your nose is not squashed and you have a sense of your neck vertebrae being in line with the rest of your spine. Your back should curve toward the floor in a long, elegant slope.

4 (*opposite*) Now anchor your right palm to the floor so that it won't slide back, and move your right hip backward to get a marvellous stretch through the whole right side of your torso. Let your chest surrender toward the floor. After ten breaths, repeat on the other side.

1

Stand with your feet about 1.5m (5ft) apart, hands on your hips. Turn your right foot out to 90 degrees and turn your left leg and foot in by 15 degrees. Square your hips, parallel to your right foot, and bend your right knee so that it sits above your right ankle.

2

Float both arms out to the side, palms down. Focus your gaze on your right middle fingertip. Slide your shoulder blades down toward your waist. Feel a line of energy running from the back of your heart along both arms to your fingertips, helping you to keep your arms horizontal.

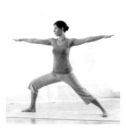

3

(*right*) Bring your right elbow to your right knee and use your elbow to push your knee slightly to the right, opening your hips. Inhale in this position, then, reaching from your left hip, extend your left arm overhead, palm facing down Turn your belly and chest upward as you gaze up and reach your left arm further over to the right.

4

Next time you inhale, swing your left arm back and raise your right arm up to bring you back to your position in step 2. Return your gaze to your right middle fingertip. Keeping your right knee at 90 degrees, exhale again to return to your side stretch. Continue for five more breaths. Then practise the whole exercise on the other side.

before
a meeting
energizing
give yourself an energy boost

1 Stand with your feet together, and hug yourself with your left arm on top. Reach so that each hand cups your opposite shoulder blade. Now move the backs of your wrists toward each other and bring your palms together. If you can't manage this, hook your top thumb with your little finger, or simply bring the backs of your wrists closer together.

2 (*right*) Bend both knees to come into a squat. Inhale and raise your right leg up. Wrap your right leg over your left thigh, and wrap your right ankle around your left calf. You'll need to keep your left knee well bent to achieve this, and hinge forward slightly at your hips.

3 If you can't wrap your right ankle fully, an alternative is to bring your right ankle to the top of your left knee. Flex your right ankle and squat deeper as you lean forward. If you find that you have trouble balancing, take small, even sips of air in and out rather than big full breaths.

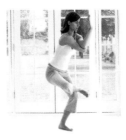

4 You can increase your shoulder stretch by lifting your elbows higher in the air, well above your chest. Increase the intensity by attempting to straighten your elbows, still intertwined. After seven breaths, release your legs and arms, reground your feet and take a couple of breaths before practising the pose on the other side.

take a
moment
focusing

bring your mind and body
back into balance

weekend sequence
invigorating

enliven your time off with flowing movements

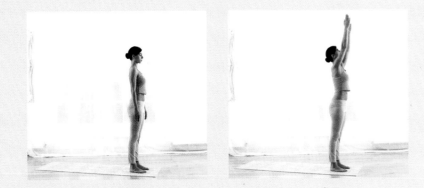

1 Ground yourself in a solid standing position with your feet hip-width apart with their outside edges parallel, and your toes pointing forward. Imagine your spine floating effortlessly tall. Allow your chest to feel buoyant. Fully relax your shoulders so your arms hang easily at your sides.

2 Inhale and reach your arms out to the sides and overhead. As you gaze up, lift your chest to create a slight backbend in your upper spine. Lift your kneecaps and keep the fronts of your thighs strong so that your lower back stays elongated.

42

3 Hinging from your hips, exhale and float your torso forward. Ensure the front of your torso stays long on this downward movement by extending forward with your chest rather than crumpling at your waist. Place your fingertips on the floor, bending your knees if necessary.

4 Inhale and step your right foot back to a lunge, so your left knee is above your left ankle. Gaze forward and lengthen your armpits away from your hips so you feel your back elongate. Keep your back leg strong by lifting the back of your right knee and extending your right ankle away from your hip.

43

weekend sequence
(continued)

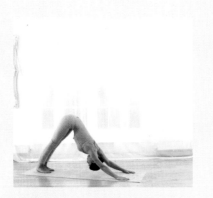

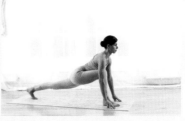

5 From your lunge position, exhale and step back so that your body is in an inverted V-shape. Ensure that your feet are hip-width apart, and your hands shoulder-width apart. Press down through your thumbs and index fingers. Extend your hips up and back, then straighten your legs and, if you are able, bring your heels to the floor.

6 As you breathe in, step your right foot between your hands. If you can't step your foot all the way forward, hook your right arm under your knee and lift your leg into your widest lunge. Come onto your fingertips and feel lighter as you extend the centre of your chest further forward.

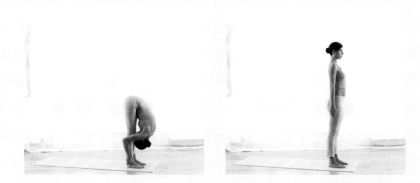

7 Exhale to step your left foot forward into a standing forward bend, keeping your torso hinged at your hips. Initially you may need to bend your knees. If you're comfortable with straight legs, intensify the stretch by tucking your chin in and grasping your ankles to draw yourself deeper into the forward bend.

8 Engage your abdominal muscles, and, on a long inhalation, bend your knees and reach your arms out to the sides to come up to standing. Exhale and lower your arms to the sides to complete the sequence. Now practise on the left side, then repeat the whole sequence four times, alternating sides.

45

before a night out
rejuvenating

revive yourself with a backbend and a forward bend

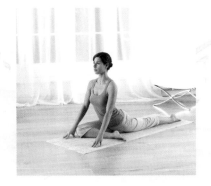 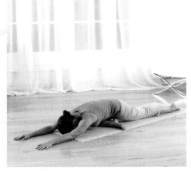

1 Start in an all-fours position. Slide your right knee toward your right wrist and move your right foot as far toward your left hand as possible – take care not to strain your knee. Place your fingertips on the floor in front of you. Use the muscles of your spine to arch into a long, even backbend and gaze straight ahead for four slow breaths.

2 Now walk your hands forward as you lower to rest your elbows on the floor. If possible, reach both arms forward to rest your forehead between them. Ease your left hip forward in space to square both hips to the front. If this is easy, move your right foot further forward, and sway your hips to the left slightly. Rest here for five breaths.

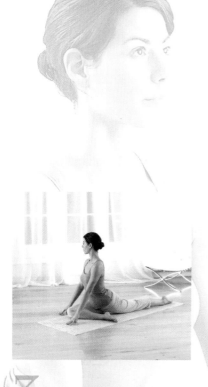

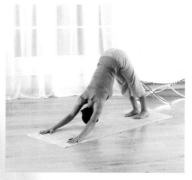

3 Bring your torso upright. Place one hand to the floor on either side of your right knee. Use your arms to lever your body into a long, strong twist. Keep your spine as vertical as possible, but take care not to compress your lower back. Activate your abdominal muscles to move them to the right. Stay here for four breaths.

4 Return your hands to centre, palms shoulder-width apart. Gently step back so that you are in an inverted V-shape. Once there, ease any knee tension by walking out your legs – alternate bending one knee while your other heel presses to the floor. Hold for five breaths. Then bring your left knee forward to practise on the other side.

47

sunday stretch
releasing

free up your body at the weekend

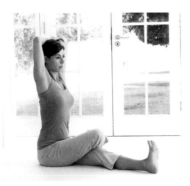
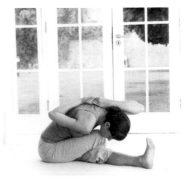

1 Sit with your legs straight out in front. Lift your right foot over your left thigh. Your right toes point out to the side. Stack your knees one on top of the other. Take your left arm overhead, thumb pointing back. Bend your elbow to bring your left hand toward your shoulder blades. Gently press your left elbow down with your right hand.

2 Reach your right arm behind you, thumb turned down. Bend your elbow to bring your hand behind your back. Catch hands, or grasp a belt between them. Roll your right shoulder back and move your elbow toward the mid-line of your body. If you are comfortable, tilt your upper body forward. Stay here for four breaths.

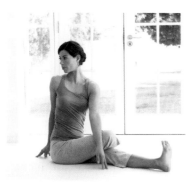
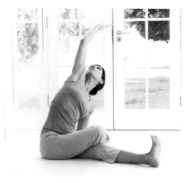

3 Gently release your arms and sit up. Keeping your chest facing the front, slide your left arm over your right thigh. Place your right hand on the floor behind you. Inhale and feel yourself grow taller. Exhaling, revolve from your lower abdomen to twist to the right, keeping your chest open. Stay here for four breaths, then release back to centre.

4 Take your left hand to the floor beside your hip. Extend your right arm in the air, thumb facing back. Inhale, lift and lengthen, then exhale and bend to the left to stretch the left side of your torso from hip to fingertips. Stay here for four breaths, then inhale back to centre, swap legs and repeat the whole exercise on the other side.

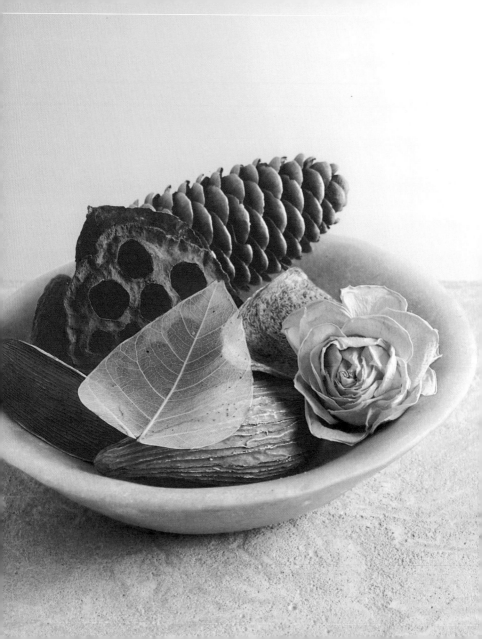

anywhere

Seize a free moment and create a space to unwind when you're feeling wound up. Be bold – after all, if you wait for conditions to be perfect, you may risk never getting started! Practise these sequences as you move through the world to bring energy, balance and relaxation to your life, whether you're at home, at work or even travelling.

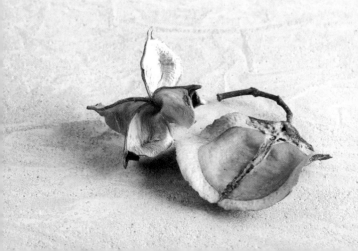

in the park
calming
find inner peace and quiet

1 (*left*) Choose a comfortable position in a quiet natural space. If you're sitting on an outdoor bench, sit up straight and place your feet hip-width apart. If you are cross-legged on the ground, sit on a gentle slope or a cushion to lift your hips higher than your knees. Rest your hands, palms-up, on your knees.

2 Close your eyes and make a mental commitment not to move your body until you have finished this exercise. Beginning from 30, start to count your breaths backward. Count so that each inhalation is one count and each exhalation is one count (30 inhale, 29 exhale, 28 inhale, 27 exhale, and so on down to 15).

3 When you reach 15, count back down to zero using only your exhalations. Pause in your counting each time you breathe in. Slowing the count down like this will help to settle a restless mind.

4 When you get to zero, stop counting and continue to watch your breath attentively, just as if you were actually still counting. You'll find the natural tendency of your mind to roam will have settled, as it is fully focused on your breathing. Stay sitting in meditation for the next couple of minutes, or longer if you can.

1 Lie comfortably on your back with your legs apart, and your hands about 15cm (6in) away from your body with your palms facing up. Close your eyes and settle into stillness. Then start to revolve your awareness around your whole body. Begin with the thumb of your right hand, then move through each finger in turn.

2 Creep your awareness up your arm to your shoulder, then to the right side of your chest, belly, hip and buttock, your right leg and foot, each of your toes and the right side of your back. Now be aware of the right side of your neck, scalp and finally the right side of your face, sensing each of your features in turn.

3 When you have completed the exercise on your right side, take a moment to notice any differences between the right and left sides of your body. You may find that your right side feels warmer, flatter, longer or just more relaxed when compared to your left.

4 Beginning with the thumb on your left hand, next rotate your awareness around the left side of your body. Take several minutes to complete this. Finally, be aware of your entire body as one. Now, feeling whole and complete, rest peacefully for as long as you wish.

on your sofa
focusing

use awareness to relax mind and body

in bed
relaxing

reset your breathing to a steady,
soothing rhythm

1 (*left*) Lie on your back with your legs 30–60cm (1–2ft) apart, feet flopping out to the sides. Check that your head is centered. Place your hands on your abdomen. This will help you to focus on your breath. Make sure that your elbows are wide and your shoulders are relaxed.

2 Close your eyes and become aware of your breathing. According to the Hatha Yoga Pradipika, an ancient yogic text, evenness of the breath promotes evenness of the mind. Regulating our breath to be smooth and steady does seem to help us navigate life's stormy seas.

3 Introduce a count to the way you are breathing. As you breathe in, count to four, and each time you breathe out, count to four. After about ten breaths, lengthen your inhalation and exhalation to a count of five. Again, after about ten breaths, add on a count, to smoothly inhale and exhale for a count of six.

4 Continue adding counts to your exhalation until you are breathing at a comfortable maximum. Some people may reach a count of eight. Make sure your breath is truly manageable; trying too hard will only create more stress on your system. When you have been counting at your maximum for ten breaths, rest and enjoy the effects of the practice.

1 Stand straight, with your feet a little wider than your hips. Ground yourself by connecting with your feet planted on the earth. To fill a vessel, first you need to empty it. Exhale and empty your lungs completely, which will make way for your fullest possible inhalation.

2 Take your arms out to the sides and up as you breathe in through your nose. This arm action will also promote a fuller inhalation. Enjoy the feeling of the sides of your ribs spreading outward and lifting, as if this expansion allows you to take more air into the sides of your lungs.

3 (*opposite*) As your arms reach up and your lungs are at their fullest, hold your breath for a moment and enjoy your full height. Bend your knees a little and, hinging at your hips and swinging your arms down and forward through your legs, flop forward and sigh out energetically through your mouth.

4 Still hanging forward with bent knees, inhale through your nose to stand and reach tall again. Complete three more cycles, sighing as loud as you want. On the exhalations, visualize letting go of something that is no longer serving you in life – for example, an old habit, an unhelpful point of view, or a cluttered mind.

58

at home
cleansing
clear your lungs and your mind

in your living room
restoring

regenerate energy whenever you are tired

1 Find a space in the middle of the floor. Fold two blankets so they are 15cm (6in) wide and a little longer than your spine. Stack them up and sit on the floor with your back facing the narrow edge of the blankets. Bring the soles of your feet together so that your knees fall out to the sides.

2 Use the cushions from your sofa, or more blankets, to pad under your knees and thighs so they receive a gentle stretch without it being too intense. This is a restorative pose you'll hold for a while and the sensations will naturally increase over time. Slowly lay your spine back along your stacked blankets.

3 Check whether you need a pillow or not: your head needs to be higher than your heart, while your chin should not be higher than your forehead. Use additional padding under your head and neck if you need to and it's comfortable.

4 (*opposite*) Rest your arms to the sides, palms face up and fingers softly curled. Allow your forearms to be heavy on the floor. Your body relaxes more completely in darkness, so close your eyes (or use an eye pillow if you prefer). Rest here, breathing deeply, for five minutes.

61

in your kitchen
releasing

enliven your whole body and release tight shoulders

1 Place your palms flat on a table or desk. Position them shoulder-width apart and spread your fingers as far apart as possible. Walk your feet back so that your ankles are under your hips. Your spine should be long and flat, like a table-top, and your body should form an L-shape.

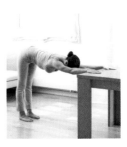

2 Work on your shoulder alignment. Your shoulders should roll out so that the outer edges of your armpits move toward each other across the front of your body. To stretch the backs of your legs more, increase the forward tilt of your pelvis by lifting your sitting bones up and away from your heels. Stay for ten long breaths, then come up and rest.

3 Now position your elbows on the edge of the table, shoulder-width apart or a little wider. Bring your palms together in prayer pose, fingers pointing to the sky. Walk your feet back as before. Increase the shoulder release by allowing your front ribs to move toward the floor.

4 (left) Pressing your palms together, slowly hinge at your elbows to lower your thumbs toward your upper back. If your shoulders are flexible, your fingertips will point toward your tailbone. Through this movement, you'll encounter a zone of increased intensity. Hold in that tight spot for ten long breaths, then come up and smile.

63

1 Sit with your right shoulder and hip next to a wall. Lean back on your palms, and walk both hands away from the wall while your elbows bend. Swivel on your buttocks to bring your legs straight up the wall, soles of the feet facing the ceiling. Lie back to rest your body on the floor.

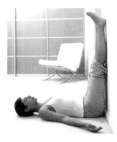

2 Once you're lying, gently lift your head to check that your legs, torso and head are in line with one another. If you're flexible, your buttocks may be close to the wall, but this pose will still work beautifully even if they're positioned a little distance away.

3 Close your eyes. Rest your arms by your side, or if it feels more luxurious, drape them in a soft halo around your head. Observe your breathing as it settles into an easy, smooth rhythm. Float restfully here for five minutes, allowing your body to sink into the floor.

4 (right) For a deeper inversion, fold two blankets to a wide wedge about 15cm (6in) high and place them 15cm (6in) from the wall. Bring your legs up the wall as before. You'll have a delightful, easy curve in your spine. Perch your tailbone over the edge of the blankets so that your abdomen is level. If you feel like you are sliding off, lower the height of the blankets. Position your arms by your sides, or over your head.

64

in a **hotel room**
reviving

rejuvenate after a long day,
or when you need some time out

at work
centering

relieve neck tension while you're working

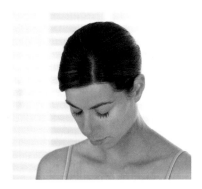 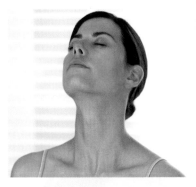

1 Choose a comfortable seated position. If you're on a chair, don't lean into the back rest. If you're cross-legged on the floor, sit on as many cushions as you need to lift your hips higher than your knees. Close your eyes to lessen distractions. Exhaling for a count of four, bend your neck, allowing your face to fall toward your lap.

2 Pause with your lungs empty for a count of two, then inhale for a count of four to bring your head back to the centre. Hold your breath in for two, then exhale for four as you lift your chin (without dropping your head so far back that it strains your neck or throat). Pause for a count of two, then inhale and bring your head back to the centre.

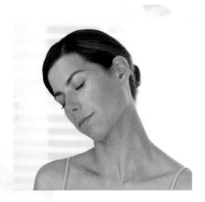

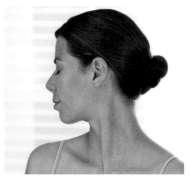

3 Working with this 4:2:4:2 breathing ratio, continue your movements for ten breaths. Then exhale and drop your right ear to your right shoulder. Pause, then inhale to return your head to centre. Hold your breath in, then repeat the movement on your left side. Pause here, then inhale back up. Repeat for ten breaths.

4 Now exhale to twist your neck and slide your chin over your right shoulder. Pause. Inhale to centre. Pause. Exhale to the left and continue, maintaining the same 4:2 breath count. After ten cycles, stop counting, sit tall and enjoy the release in your neck and the quietness in your mind. When you feel ready, open your eyes.

at your desk energizing

invigorate yourself during a long day at work

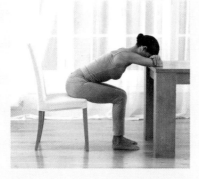 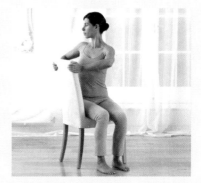

1 Sitting with your feet and knees about 60cm (2ft) apart, move your chair 60–90cm (2–3ft) away from your desk. Lay your forearms on the edge of your desk and rest your forehead on them. Use your back muscles to drop your abdomen and chest toward the floor. With your back turned on the world, breathe 15 full breaths.

2 Sit sideways on your chair with your feet hip-width apart. Inhale and allow your spine to float tall, then exhale and twist to grasp the back of the chair, with your hands wide. With each inhalation, grow taller. With each exhalation, spiral deeper into the twist. After eight long breaths, change sides.

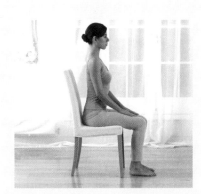

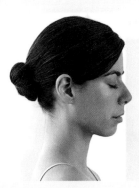

3 Sit upright so that the natural curves of your spine are intact, rather than leaning against the back of your chair. Sense your head balancing easily at the top of your spine. Rest your hands on your thighs so that your elbows hang relaxed, loose and free, just below your shoulder joints.

4 Close your eyes and become aware of your breath. Notice how your body moves one way to let the air in, and another way to let it out. With every inhalation, just "know" that you are breathing in. With every exhalation, just "know" that you are breathing out. Stay here for 20 breaths, or longer if you have time.

at your computer
soothing
give screen-tired eyes a break

1 Sit comfortably, cross-legged or on a chair. First, exercise the small muscles that control your eyeballs. Move both eyeballs as far as you can to the left. Then move them horizontally, all the way to the right. Repeat ten times in each direction. Then close your eyes and rest.

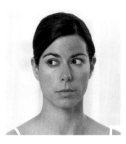

2 Next, work vertically. Keeping your head centered, look up as far as you can. Then gaze downward as far a possible. Try not to move your head up and down; isolate just your eye muscles to move them independently. Repeat ten times, then close your eyes and rest.

3 Now move your eyes in circles. Roll your eyeballs up and rotate them in a clockwise direction. Be sure to move them in slow, generous circles with no flat edges. After five circles, close your eyes and rest. Then repeat the circles, rotating anti-clockwise five times.

4 (*left*) Rub your palms together, using the friction to create as much warmth as you can manage. Close your eyes, and cover them with your palms. Breathe deeply and enjoy the warm darkness. Some people find a light palm pressure on their eyelids even more soothing. Stay here for eight breaths, then release any pressure, cup your palms, blink your eyes open underneath them, then slowly lower your hands.

71

1 (*opposite*) Sit with your eyes closed. Take a few breaths to settle yourself. Begin this meditation by directing compassion to yourself. In your mind repeat several times "May I be happy, safe and well." If this feels difficult, imagine yourself as a small child in need of love and protection. Send loving kindness to this child within.

2 Now that you've extended loving kindness to yourself, you'll be ready to send it out to others, too. Visualize someone you love. Holding that person in your heart, send them loving kindness. Allow your heart to open as you repeat "May you be happy, safe and well."

3 Now think of someone who represents a challenge in your life. Although you may find it more difficult to hold this person in your heart, direct loving kindness to them. Wish this person well on their path as you develop your compassion, repeating several times "May you be happy, safe and well."

4 Now send loving kindness to everyone around you. Repeat "May you all be happy, safe and well." Expand this circle of compassion to include all living beings: "May all beings be happy, safe and well." Finally, bring your awareness back to yourself. Be aware of the pleasant expanded feeling in your heart. Blink your eyes open, and continue with your day.

on a **train**
uplifting

develop your compassion
to connect with the world

on a plane
energizing

re-energize and restore in-flight

1 (*left*) Sit upright in your plane seat; leaning back will inhibit the freedom of your lungs. Place your right palm on your chest and your left palm on your abdomen. Close your eyes. This practice encourages a full expansion of your lungs, which is tremendously energizing, while the slow emptying of your lungs is very calming.

2 Exhale to begin. Breathe in until your lungs are about one-third full. Pause for two counts. Breathe in until they are two-thirds full. Pause for two counts. Breathe in again until your lungs are completely full. Hold your breath in for two counts.

3 Release the air in one smooth, unhurried exhalation. Take a couple of normal breaths to recover. Repeat these stepped inhalations twice more. Notice how your abdomen and chest each move in response to the slow and complete filling of the lungs.

4 Exhale normally, then inhale in one slow, deep continuous breath. Hold your breath in for two counts, then exhale to empty one third out. Pause for two counts, then exhale another third. Pause, then exhale to completely empty your lungs. Pause with empty lungs for two counts. Take a few normal breaths to recover, then repeat the exhalations twice more.

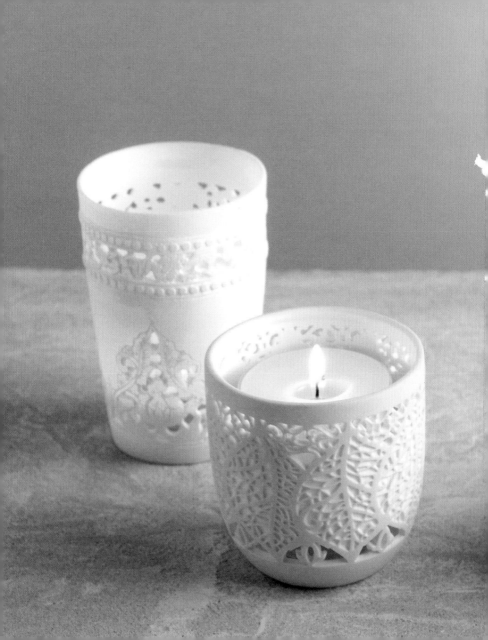

stress
busters

To counter tension in mind or body, completely absorb yourself in

any one of these practices. Journey inward, and focus fully on the

sensations of your body. If you can turn away from those everyday

worries and go within for even just one minute, you'll feel a gratifying

shift in your inner world, and re-emerge fresh and focused.

tension reliever
releasing

soften and release tight shoulders

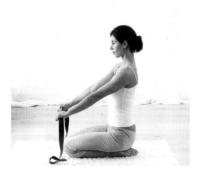
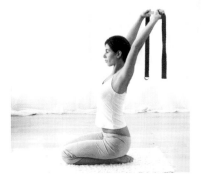

1 Kneel with your heels under your buttocks, or sit cross-legged. Grasp a soft belt in front of you with your hands about 1m (3¼ft) apart. Inhale and raise both arms overhead. Exhale and move your arms in an arc, to take them behind your back.

2 Inhale and raise your hands once again; then exhale as you bring them in front of you. Continue the movements, all the way back and forth, for ten more breaths. Time your movements with your breath. If you find a particularly tight spot, hold your arms there and inhale and exhale a few times, allowing space for softening to occur.

3 Put the belt aside and reach your right arm overhead, turning your thumb to point behind you. Bend your right elbow to take your right hand down your back. Grasp your right elbow with your left hand, and ease your right arm toward the centre line of the back of your head. Breathe.

4 Keeping your right arm in place, drop your left hand by your side. Rotating from your shoulder joint, turn your left thumb behind you. Bend your elbow to catch hands (or hold the belt between your hands if you can't reach). Stay here for ten breaths, then practise on the other side. Release and notice the relaxation in your shoulders.

body calmer
relaxing

clear your mind, just like magic

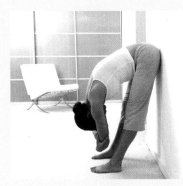 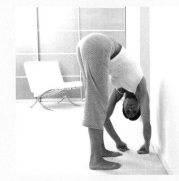

1 Stand with your back against a wall. Take your feet hip-width apart, about 30cm (12in) from the wall. Hinge forward from your hips. Hold your elbows and just hang for eight breaths. Release the muscles of your neck and shoulders. Slide your sitting bones higher up the wall, or, if you need to soften the intensity, bend your knees.

2 If your back feels pleasantly long and flat, try this more challenging variation. Turn around and position your toes 45cm (18in) away from the wall. Check that the outer edges of your feet are parallel. Sway to one side and fold forward. With your hands on the floor, walk your feet toward the wall to bring your upper back against the wall.

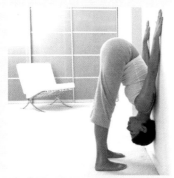

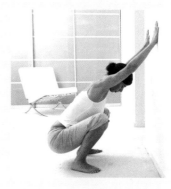

3 Still using your hands as support, Lean your hips strongly toward the wall to help your shoulder blades slide lower down the wall. Keep your heels grounded and your knees straight. Try to have your hip joints in front of your ankle joints. If possible, rotate your shoulder joints to plant both palms high up the wall. Stay here for eight breaths.

4 Bring your hands to the floor to steady yourself. Turn toward the wall if you need to, and turn your toes and knees out an equal amount. Drop your hips to a squat, with your heels lifted if that is more comfortable. Bring your palms to the wall, and take some time to settle the effects of the inversion before slowly standing up.

81

1 Lie on your front, with your forehead on the floor. Tuck in your chin to lengthen the back of your neck and ensure you can breathe easily through your nose. Activate your legs to create a current of energy running down the fronts of your legs to your toes. Maintain this leg action during the whole of the following exercise.

2 Place your palms so that your fingertips are level with your shoulders. Root your thumbs and index fingers to the floor. Slide your shoulder blades toward your waist and peel your chest off the floor. Keep your shoulders rolling back and down, your elbows slightly bent and tucked in toward your side-ribs, and your neck in line with your spine.

3 (*right*) Maintain firm back muscles, almost as if your arms were not there to support you. Gaze up, straight ahead or to the floor. Fully involve yourself in the intensity of the pose by pressing your chestbone forward and up. Stay here for eight breaths, and repeat twice.

4 Move your feet and knees together and sit back on your heels. Lay your ribs over your thighs and rest your forehead on the floor. Drape your arms alongside your body. Relax here for at least two minutes, breathing mindfully.

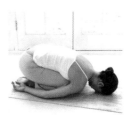

focus booster
centering
move your awareness into the present moment

back reliever
unwinding

bring vitality and positivity to your day

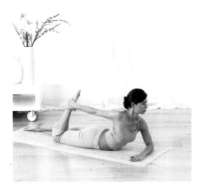 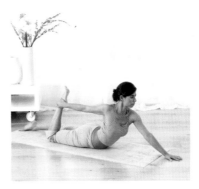

1 Lie down on your front, and prop yourself up on your elbows, palms on the floor. Bend your right knee and reach your right arm back to grasp your ankle. Press your right leg away as if you wanted to straighten it, and lift your chest into a long, even backbend. Direct the right side of your ribcage forward to stop yourself twisting to the right.

2 If you can go further, slide your left hand forward and straighten your elbow. Don't hunch your left shoulder – keep it rolling back and down. Lift your chest high and focus on the arch in your upper and mid-back. Hold for six breaths. Now repeat the whole exercise with your left knee bent.

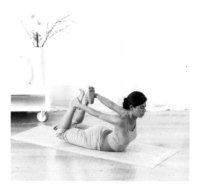

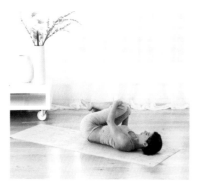

3 For the full pose, lie on the floor and grasp both feet. Press both legs away and lift your upper body high. Keep your elbows straight and develop the arch in your upper back by squeezing your shoulder blades together. As you breathe strongly, you will rock gently backward and forward. Hold for eight breaths and repeat twice more.

4 Roll onto your back and hug your knees into your chest. Squeeze them in and rock slowly from side to side to ease any tension out of your back. Then, cup your right knee in your right hand, and your left knee in your left hand, and enjoy making six slow circling movements, three clockwise and then three anti-clockwise.

85

1 Stand, feet together, hands on hips. Step your right leg about 50cm (1½ft) behind you, bringing the tips of your toes to the floor. Energize through your back leg and press your chest upward to create a crescent moon shape with your body. Roll your shoulders back to bring your elbows toward each other. Allow your chest to feel lifted.

2 Press your right hip forward to square your hips to the front. Hinging at the top of your left thigh, bend forward as you simultaneously extend through your right leg to lift it off the floor, heel pointed to the ceiling. Maintain the arched shape of your back as you bring your torso and leg to a long line parallel with the floor.

3 If your right hip has lifted, correct this by dropping your hip so that your lower back is flat – imagine a glass of water balancing in the centre of your lower back. If this is difficult, bend your supporting leg. To help you balance, gaze at a single point about 90cm (3ft) in front of you.

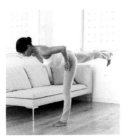

4 (*right*) To reach the full pose, strengthen your abdominal muscles and extend your arms out, palms facing each other, parallel to the floor. Activate your back muscles more. Breathe and balance here for five breaths. Then come out and practise on the other side.

all over re-balancer

steadying

develop your mental and physical poise

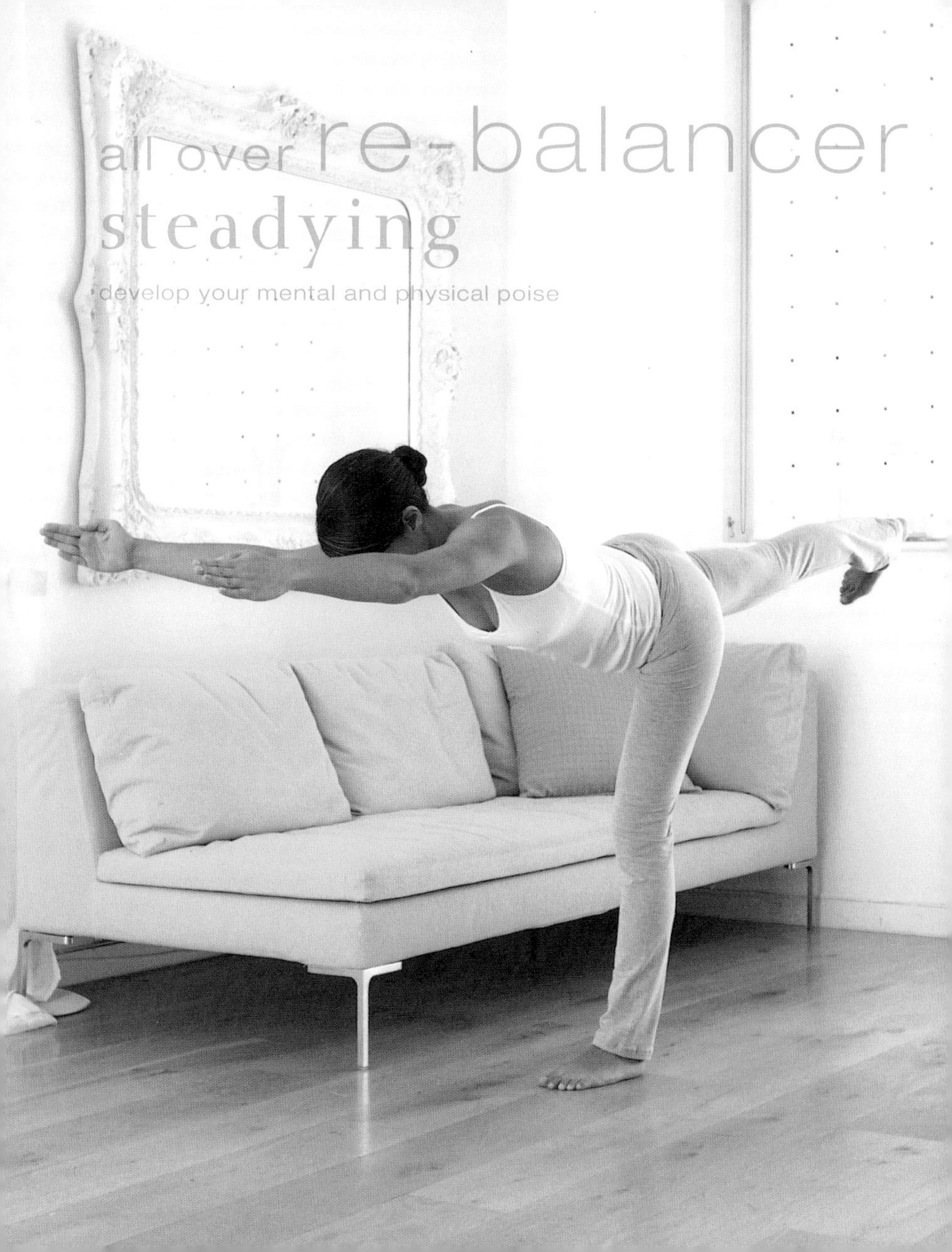

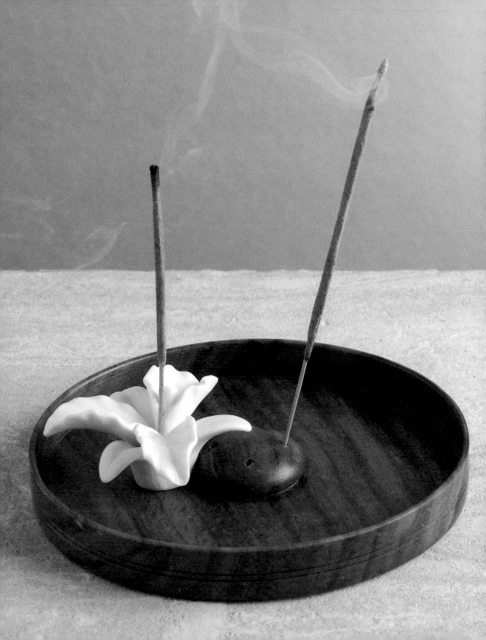

mood enhancers

Don't put off feeling happy — use the tried-and-tested techniques of yoga to feel better today! Our bodies were designed to move and stretch, and they love it. Allow the postures in this chapter to unblock pent-up physical tensions, and combine them with deep rhythmic breathing to calm and soothe a troubled mind.

core reviver
releasing

steady your breath to help steady your mind and mood

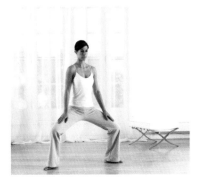 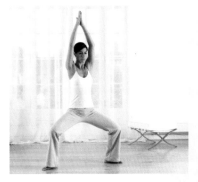

1 Place your feet 90cm (3ft) apart, or wider if you have long legs. Turn your toes out to 45 degrees. Bend your knees over your ankles so that you are in a wide-legged squat. Ensure that your knees are tracking in the same direction as your toes. Rest your palms on your thighs and take a moment to notice how you are feeling.

2 Bring your arms by your sides and turn your palms out. Inhale and reach your arms out and up until your palms join overhead. Move at a constant rate, and time this action to a mental count of four. Once your palms are together, exhale and bring them down through the mid-line of your body, again to the mental count of four.

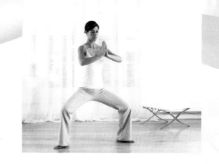

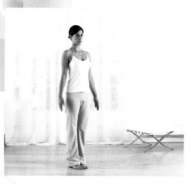

3 Continue to breathe while moving your arms out, up and down at a constant, flowing rate. Enjoy the feeling of inhaling your breath deeply into your lungs and the sides of your ribcage. Each time you exhale and lower your palms, imagine that the downward movement of your arms is helping to push the air out of your lungs.

4 If you can comfortably move and breathe more slowly, count five or six rather than four. Continue for 15 breaths, then step your legs together and stand tall. Check in with yourself. How is your body feeling now? How has this practice altered your mood?

CORE REVIVER

1 Lie on your back and hug your knees in to your chest. Press your thighs against your abdomen to help empty your lungs as you exhale. Ease off and notice your belly and chest expanding toward your thighs as you inhale. Allow your breath to settle into a smooth rhythm.

2 Place your feet on the floor hip-width apart. Slowly inhale, extend your arms overhead and lift your hips. Lift the fronts of your thighs as high as possible. Broaden your shoulders on the floor.

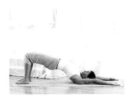

3 (*right*) On your next exhalation, lower your hips to the floor and bring your knees to your chest once more. Allow your tailbone to lift. Cup your hands over your knees and squeeze your thighs in again. Exhale completely, to make space for a much deeper inhalation.

4 Inhale and extend your legs up into the air as your arms flow up and over your head once more. If this leg movement feels too strong in your hamstrings or lower back, take care to bend your knees

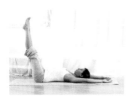

slightly when your legs are overhead. Exhale and hug your knees in to your chest again and practise the whole sequence seven times.

breath soother
uplifting

loosen your shoulders and strengthen your core

body invigorator
heartening

bring yourself back into re-energized balance

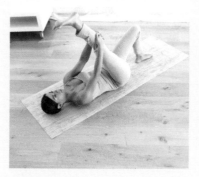 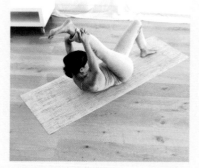

1 Lie on your back with your right leg stretched straight in the air. Your left knee should be bent, with the sole of the foot on the floor. Interlace your fingers behind your right thigh or calf, and gently pull your leg toward your torso for eight breaths. Intensify the stretch by flexing your ankle, to aim your toes toward your head.

2 Tuck in your chin and lift your head toward your knee. If you can, walk your hands higher up your leg, and exhale to deepen the stretch. Resist bending your knee and move your knee even closer to your head. Stay here for six breaths. Keeping your leg in the air, exhale and release your head to the floor, and your arms out to the sides.

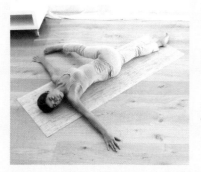 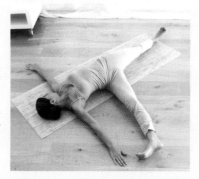

3 Straighten your left leg. Inhale, then exhale and take your right foot over to the left, toward the floor. If possible, point your right toes toward your left hand. Stack your right hip on top of your left as you twist your neck to turn your head to the right.

4 Inhale and bring your right leg up to vertical, then exhale and take your right foot toward the floor near your right hand. Turn your head to the left. Repeat this side-to-side cycle for four breaths, inhaling your leg up to a vertical position, and exhaling it to the side. Then practise the whole exercise from the beginning with your left leg.

heart lifter
stabilizing

blow your cares away with this classic backbend

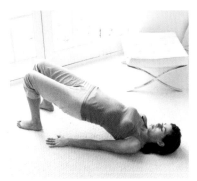 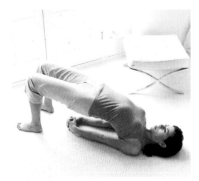

1 Lie on your back with your arms by your sides, palms facing down. Bend your knees and place your feet on the floor, hip-width apart. Inhale, and beginning from your tailbone and moving up your spine, slowly raise your hips up and toward your knees. Hold this position for six slow, deep breaths, then release down to rest.

2 Lift your hips as before, then tilt to your right and roll your left shoulder down and under your chest. Tip left to repeat the movement with your right shoulder. Interlace your fingers and reach them toward your heels, elbows straight. Hold this pose for six breaths, enjoying the shoulder stretch. Release your hands and rest down.

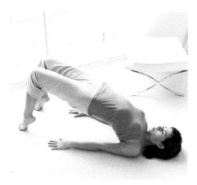 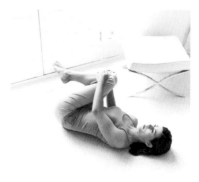

3 This enjoyable modification allows more elongation in your lower back. Lift your hips as high as you can and roll your shoulders under as in step 2. Lift your heels so that you are on tiptoes, and move your chestbone toward your chin. Remain on tiptoes and take a full minute to lower your back, vertebrae by vertebrae, to the floor.

4 Finish with a self-administered back massage. Hug your knees in to your chest and roll from side to side to release tension in your entire back. If you're on a soft surface, move your knees away from your chest a little and try rocking backward and forward.

1 Sit erect, cross-legged or on a chair. Ensure that your nostrils are clear. Bring the index and middle fingers of your left hand in toward your palm. You will use your ring finger, little finger and thumb to close each nostril in turn. If you prefer, you can use your right hand instead.

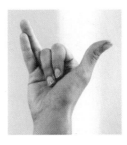

2 (*right*) Using your left ring and little fingers, cover your right nostril. Breathe out through your left nostril. Then inhale through it. Cover your left nostril with your thumb. Release your ring and little fingers and exhale through your right nostril. Then inhale through it.

3 Repeat this sequence, changing nostrils after each inhalation. Close your eyes and keep your breath smooth and even. Imagine a thin silver thread of air flowing leisurely in and out of each nostril. Allow time for the natural pauses that separate your inhalations and exhalations.

4 Take care to keep your left shoulder relaxed and your head centered. When you have completed ten breaths, lower your arm and stay seated with your eyes closed. Notice how you are feeling now. This is a beautiful practice for first thing in the morning, or before bed, or for any time that you need to find a moment of peace during the day.

breath
balancer
calming

master this practice to alter your mood

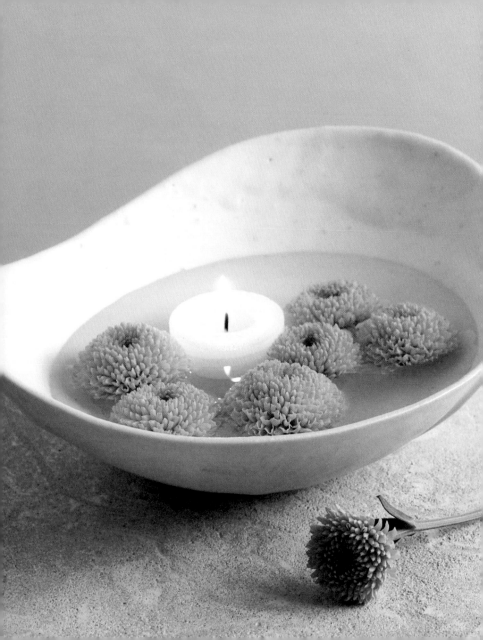

energy
boosters

Using all your muscle strength to stretch deeply in a yoga sequence can actually give you more energy. Give any one of these sequences all you've got and you'll reap generous rewards. The poses in this chapter will leave you feeling open, fresh and vibrant.

energy enhancer strengthening

work your entire body to refresh your whole system

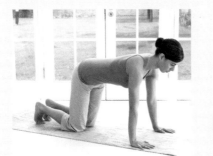 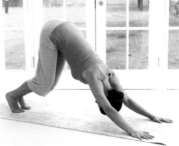

1 Begin in an all-fours position, with your knees and feet hip-width apart. Place your hands shoulder-width apart so that your middle fingers point forward. Press down evenly through your palms, with particular attention to maintaining firm pressure through your thumb and index finger.

2 Lift your hips up and back so that your legs and back form an inverted V-shape, with your knees bent. Roll your shoulders outward to create plenty of space between your upper arms and your neck – imagine that you have eyeballs in your armpits and they are going cross-eyed across your chest.

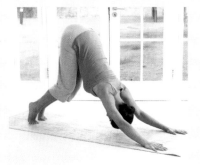 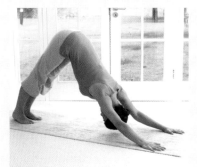

3 Next, lift your heels and bend your knees deeply. Ease your chest toward the fronts of your thighs, creating a ski-jump shape with your spine. Continue to spread your shoulder blades apart, resisting the urge to hunch your shoulders, and maintain a firm pressure on the whole of your palm.

4 Now involve the backs of your legs. Work toward straightening them, moving your heels toward the floor. If they reach the floor, walk your feet backward. Keep working your back toward an arch shape. Stay for ten long breaths before resting on all fours.

strength builder
enlivening

develop strength and firmness in your upper body

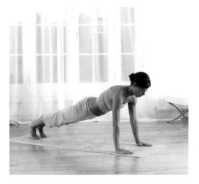
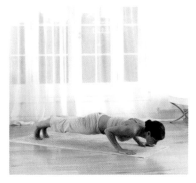

1 Begin in an all-fours position, with your middle fingers facing forward. Tuck your toes under and lift your knees. Walk your feet back so that the back of your body forms a straight line from shoulders to heels, with your shoulders above your wrists and your buttocks in line. Check that the creases of your inner elbows face forward.

2 Engage your abdominal strength by drawing your lower ribs toward your hipbones. Exhale, and bend your elbows to lower your body to hover just above the ground. Your elbows should stay snug to the sides of your ribs, rather than splaying wide. If you need to build strength first, you can lower your knees to the floor.

104

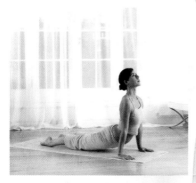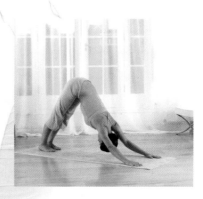

3 Inhale and press your chest forward between your upper arms while straightening your elbows. Simultaneously, roll forward over the tips of your toes to rest on the fronts of your feet. Maintain plenty of energy in the fronts of your legs so that your kneecaps don't sag toward the floor.

4 Exhale, and draw your navel toward your spine to engage your abdominals as you move into an inverted V-shape. Roll backward over your toes as you lift your hips up and back. Press down through your heels to lengthen the backs of your legs. Inhale to come forward to the position in step 1. Repeat the whole sequence five times.

back refresher opening

enliven the front of your body with a backbend

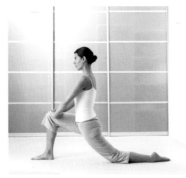

1 From a kneeling position, step your right foot forward. Bend your right knee to a position just above your ankle and slide your hips forward. Place your hands on your right knee. Tuck your tailbone under to deepen the stretch in the front of your left thigh.

2 Lean forward slightly to elongate your lower back. Reach both arms forward and, inhaling deeply, extend them vertically. Have your palms facing toward each other to encourage your shoulder blades to spread, and to eliminate any hunching.

106

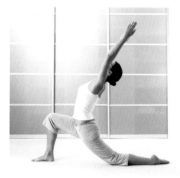

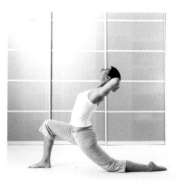

3 Reach upward with your arms and stretch up along the sides of your torso. Visualize pockets of blue sky between each of your vertebrae. If you wish, move your upper arms back and gaze upward while lifting your chest to come into a full backbend. Hold this posture for six breaths.

4 If your neck feels like it would benefit from more support, interlace your fingers behind your head. While your chest lifts upward, spread your elbows further apart and ease them back. Hold this pose for five to ten breaths. Then repeat the whole sequence with your left foot in front.

1

Kneel with both your legs bent round to the left, and your right calf tucked under your left thigh. It's natural to lean to the right a little, but if you feel like you're tipping heavily, place a blanket folded into a wedge 15cm (6in) thick underneath your right buttock.

2

Bring your left hand to the outside of your right knee. Take your right fingertips to the floor behind you. Experiment with the position of this hand to give you effective leverage into the twist. Check that you're not leaning sideways or backward·and keep your head centered.

3

Inhale and lift your chest. Exhaling, rotate from the base of your spine to twist toward the right. Gaze over your right shoulder. Hold for eight breaths, then turn your head to look over your left shoulder. Hold for four breaths. Turn your knees to the right and repeat on the other side.

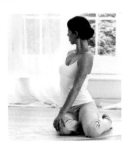

4

(*right*) If you find this exercise easy, come into the twist again and slide your right hand behind your back to grasp your left upper arm. Lean forward and grasp your right knee with your left hand. Twist to the right, and allow the right side of your chest to revolve more with each exhalation. Stay here for four breaths, and repeat on the other side.

body reviver
invigorating
refresh your body and revitalize your mind

life-force booster
rejuvenating

dynamically increase your strength and vitality

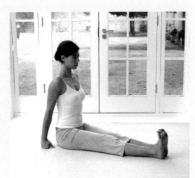 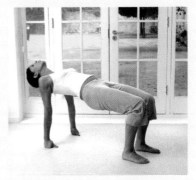

1 Sit on the floor with your legs straight out in front. Make fists with your hands, and take them to the floor just behind your buttocks. Flex your ankles to pull your toes back toward your trunk. Send strengthening energy through your arms and press your shoulders away from your ears.

2 Bend your knees and slide your hips forward and up, so that the soles of your feet come to the floor and your body forms a table-like shape. Consciously lengthen through your arms. Choose the most comfortable position for your neck: looking forward to your knees or upward to the sky.

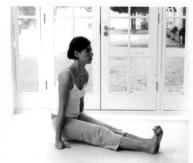

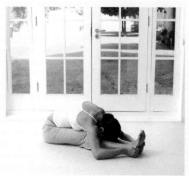

3 Exhale and lower your hips while straightening your legs. Hover your buttocks just above the floor behind your fists. Inhale and bend your knees to once again float your hips up and forward. Exhale down to hover again, and inhale back up to hold. Inhale up and exhale down four more times.

4 Now stretch out the back of your body with a forward bend. Sitting with both legs straight out in front, tilt from your pelvis and fold forward. Depending on your flexibility, grasp your thighs, calves or feet and stay here for eight full, deep breaths, moving your ribcage forward on each exhalation.

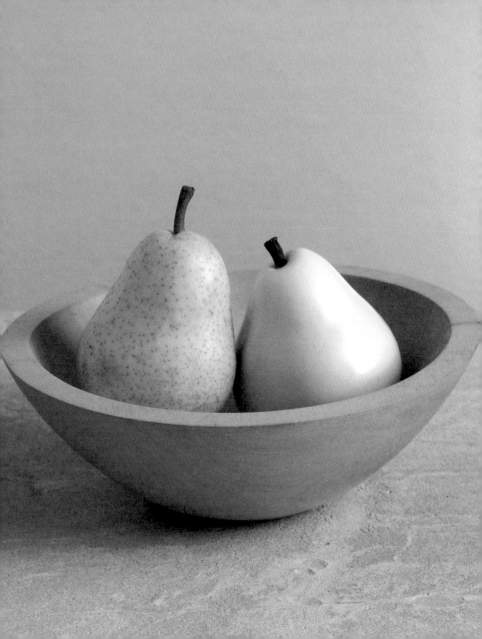

practising together

Firm a friendship and develop awareness and sensitivity with this shared practice. Working with a partner means that you can stretch more deeply, while breathing together is bonding and heart-opening. Enjoy strength and suppleness in tandem with a trusted friend.

breath connector balancing

free up your breath and mobilize your shoulders and torso

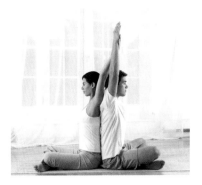

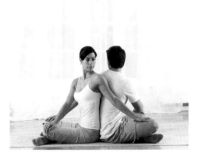

1 Sit cross-legged, back-to-back with your partner. Take your arms out to the sides, cross your wrists over your partner's, and bring your palms to your partner's palms or wrists. As you both inhale, bring your arms overhead, with bent elbows if necessary. Lower them down in time with your exhalation. Repeat this cycle ten times.

2 Return to sitting cross-legged. Grasp your left knee with your right hand, twist to the left and reach your left hand behind to grasp your partner's right knee. Breathe together. Inhale and feel yourselves grow taller, exhale and use your hands to ease deeper into the twist. Hold this position for five breaths, then repeat on the other side.

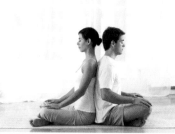

3 Position your arms wide again, with your wrists crossed. As you inhale, bring one pair of arms up into the air. Exhale to slide the other pair of hands along the floor to come into a long side stretch. Hold for five breaths. Then repeat on the other side.

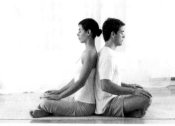

4 Return to your starting position, and place your hands on your own knees. Check that you are mutually helping each other to sit tall. Close your eyes and breathe mindfully for two minutes. Be aware of your back expanding toward your partner's with each inhalation, and use this as a tool to help you stay focused on your breath.

stamina builder
energizing

invigorate and energize with the help of a partner

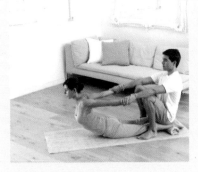 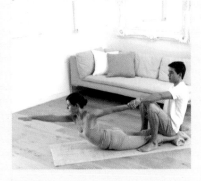

1 Lie face-down with your legs together, your arms by your sides and some padding such as a rolled-up towel under your ankles. Ask your partner to sit on your ankles, facing your head. Lift your head and chest off the floor, and reach back to grasp wrists with your partner. Stay here for four breaths, then rest down.

2 Grasp wrists with your partner again, and rise up into your long strong backbend. Once you are at your maximum height, release your right arm forward and straight out. Your partner should keep his or her gripping arm straight by leaning back and taking his or her right hand to the floor. After four breaths, change arms, then rest.

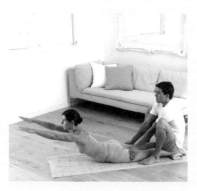

3 Lift up again with the help of your partner and, when you are ready, release both arms forward and up. Continue to work your back muscles strongly while directing your chestbone forward. Stay here for four breaths, then grasp wrists behind you again. Allow your partner to help you lift as high as you can, before resting down.

4 Sit back on your heels and bring your forehead to the floor. Ask your partner to place one hand on your mid-back and the other at the base of your spine, and press down with both hands while moving them apart. Enjoy this relaxing position for a full minute, then swap over so that your partner can practise the whole exercise.

117

limbering hip
opener
mobilizing

have fun bonding with a friend
during some deep stretches

1 Sit opposite your partner with the soles of your own feet together and your toes touching your partner's. Grasp each other's wrists or forearms. Allow your spines to elongate, and your knees to widen. Start to rotate your upper bodies in large clockwise circles. Ensure that each circle lasts for one full breath.

2 Be sure that you're not rotating from your ribcage; drop your energy into your pelvis and move from here. Create smooth, generous circles, with no flat edges. Allow yourself time to be aware of your movement, and use the backward arc as an abdominal strengthener. After ten circles, change direction.

3 (left) Return to your starting position. Inhale and float your chests upward, then exhale to stretch forward as your partner leans back. Inhale to return to centre, then exhale to swap positions. Continue this flow for ten breaths, inhaling to return to centre, then exhaling as each of you leans back in turn.

4 Now stay in the forward bend for eight breaths. Enjoy a sense of lengthening through the sides of your waist. If you're very flexible in this forward movement, you may need to hold higher up each other's arms. The person leaning back will be building abdominal strength. Swap over, then rest.

1 (*right*) Sit back-to-back with your partner, with your legs straight out in front. Inhale and feel yourselves grow taller. Exhale and fold forward as your partner simultaneously lays back along your spine, his or her weight encouraging you into a deep forward bend. Depending on your flexibility, bring your hands to your thighs, shins or feet. If you feel the stretch is too intense as you bend forward, bend your knees a little.

2 On the next inhalation, you and your partner return to the starting position. On the next exhalation, swap positions, so that your partner is bending forward. Repeat for four breaths, continuing to flow into these forward bends and backbends by inhaling up and exhaling down.

3 Once you are warm, hold in each position for up to two minutes. The extra time will allow both of you to settle your breathing as you ease deeper into the postures. The forward-bending partner will feel a strong stretch along the whole back of their body.

4 While you are enjoying the passive backbend, connect with a full expansion of your chest with each inhalation. Let your arms be heavy and your hands rest on the floor, fingers softly curled. If your chin is higher than your forehead, use some soft padding under your head.

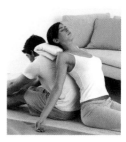

back soother opening

drop into wonderfully relaxing forward bends

body balancer releasing

loosen up your hips, thighs and torso

1   Sit with your legs wide apart, with your feet between your partner's legs. Allow your pelvis to rotate forward a little so that you are sitting on the front edges of your buttock bones. If you feel yourself slouching backward, bend both knees to allow your spine to lift with less effort.

2   (*left*) Grasp your partner's wrists. Inhale and lengthen through your waist as you grow taller. As you exhale, stretch forward as your partner leans back. Inhale to return to centre, and exhale to swap positions. Continue to flow, inhaling up to centre and exhaling down for ten breaths, then each of you hold the forward bend for eight breaths.

3   With your partner easing you forward, this is strong, deep work. If you are very flexible, you may need to hold each other's elbows so that the backward-moving partner isn't too low for comfort. Feel that your spine is becoming flatter with each exhalation.

4   Now grasp your partner's right wrist with your right hand. Lift both left arms in the air and bend to the right to give your left sides a long stretch. Feel a line of energy moving from your left hip through to your fingertips. After six slow breaths, repeat this stretch on the other side.

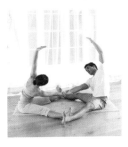

everyday sequences

Try out these simple yoga sequences whenever you have a little more time. If your selected exercise is shown at a particular time or place (for example, at work or on your sofa), bear in mind that you can practise at any time, in any suitable location.

half-hour unwinder	half-hour calmer	half-hour stabilizer
78 tension reliever	94 body invigorator	90 core reviver
30 afternoon stabilizer	48 sunday stretch	22 morning activator
106 back refresher	36 close the day	38 before a meeting
92 breath soother	34 bedtime wind-down	40 take a moment
60 in your living room	98 breath balancer	96 heart lifter
56 in bed	54 on your sofa	80 body calmer

index

acknowledgments

publisher's acknowledgments

The publisher wou[...]   modelling, Nicky West for
consulting on the y[...]   an for the models' hair and
make-up, and Adam Giles for assisting with the photography.